Plant-Based Cookbook

The Importance of Choosing a Sustainable Alimentation

The Green Solution

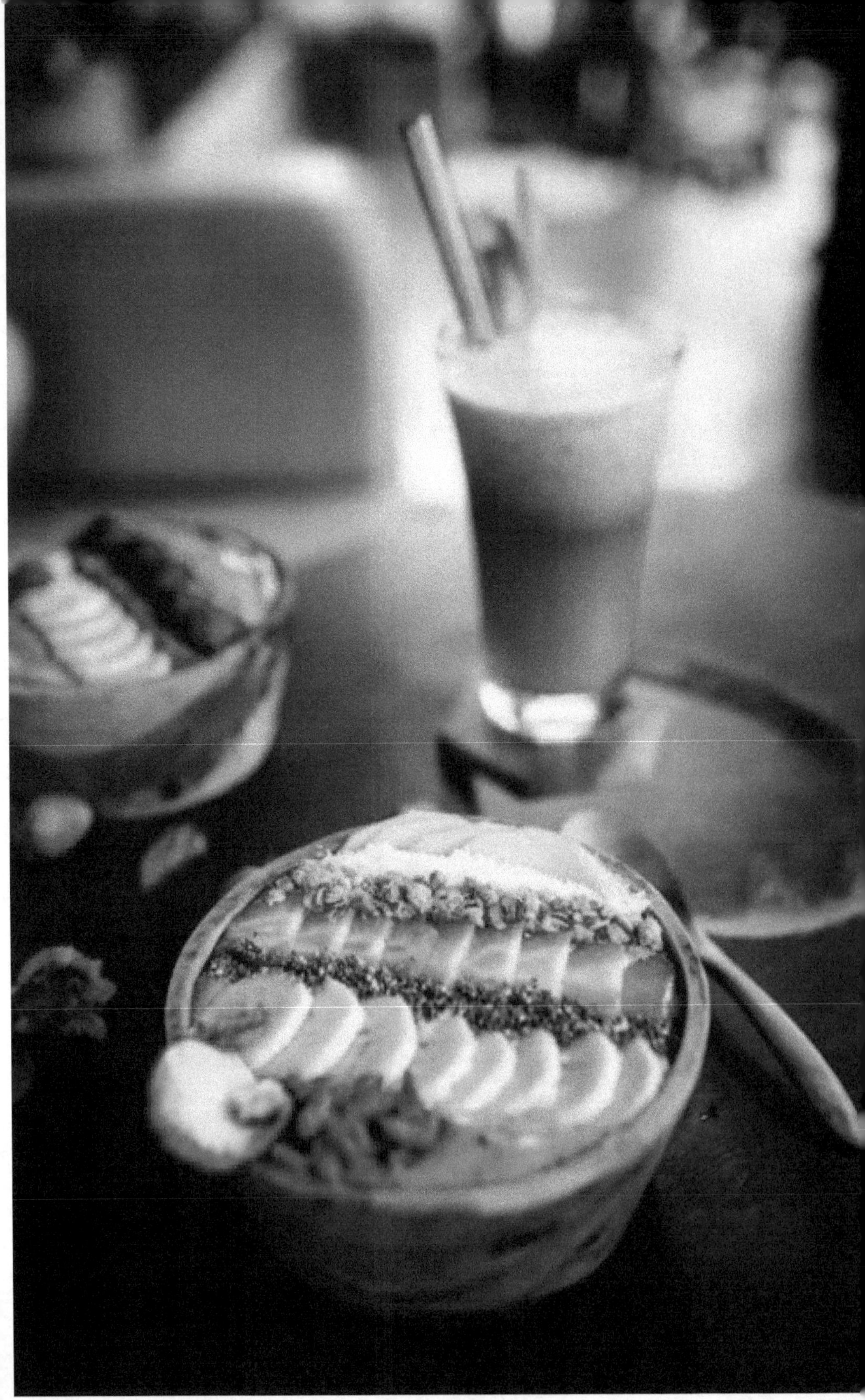

Additionally, the information in the following pages is intended only for informational purposes and should thus be thought of as universal. As befitting its nature, it is presented without assurance regarding its prolonged validity or interim quality. Trademarks that are mentioned are done without written consent and can in no way be considered an endorsement from the trademark holder.

Table of Contents

INTRODUCTION

A plant-based diet is a diet consisting mostly or entirely of plant-based foods with no animal products or artificial ingredients. While a plant-based diet avoids or has limited animal products, it is not necessarily vegan. This includes not only fruits and vegetables, but also nuts, seeds, oils, whole grains, legumes, and beans. It doesn't mean that you are vegetarian or vegan and never eat meat, eggs, or dairy.

Vegetarian diets have also been shown to support health, including a lower risk of developing coronary heart disease, high blood pressure, diabetes, and increased longevity.

Plant-based diets offer all the necessary carbohydrates, vitamins, protein, fats, and minerals for optimal health, and are often higher in fiber and phytonutrients. However, some vegans may need to add a supplement to ensure they receive all the nutrients required.

Who says that plant-based diets are limited or boring? There are lots of delicious recipes that you can use to make mouthwatering, healthy, plant-based dishes that will satisfy your cravings. If you're eating these plant-based foods regularly, you can maintain a healthy weight without obsessing about calories and avoid diseases that result from bad dietary habits.

Benefits of a Plant-Based Diet

Eating a plant-based diet improves the health of your gut so you are better able to absorb the nutrients from food that support your immune system and reduce inflammation. Fiber can lower cholesterol and stabilize blood sugar, and it's great for good bowel management.

- **A Plant-Based Diet May Lower Your Blood Pressure**
  High blood pressure, or hypertension, can increase the risk for health issues, including heart disease, stroke, and type 2 diabetes and reduce blood pressure and other risky conditions.

- **A Plant-Based Diet May Keep Your Heart Healthy**
  Saturated fat in meat can contribute to heart issues when eaten in excess, so plant-based foods can help keep your heart healthy.

- **A Plant-Based Diet May Help Prevent Type 2 Diabetes**
  Animal foods can increase cholesterol levels, so eating a plant-based diet filled with high-quality plant foods can reduce the risk of developing type 2 diabetes by 34 percent.

- **Eating a Plant-Based Diet Could Help You Lose Weight**
  Cutting back on meat can help you to maintain a healthy weight because a plant-based diet is naturally satisfying and rich in fiber.

- **Following a Plant-Based Diet Long Term May Help You Live Longer**
  If you stick with healthy plant-based foods your whole body will be leaner and healthier, allowing you to stay healthy and vital as you age.

- **A Plant-Based Diet May Decrease Your Risk of Cancer**
  Vegetarians have an 18 percent lower risk of cancer compared to non-vegetarians. This is because a plant-based diet is rich of fibers and healthy nutrients.

- **A Plant-Based Diet May Improve Your Cholesterol**
  High cholesterol can lead to fatty deposits in the blood, which can restrict blood flow and potentially lead to heart attack, stroke, heart disease, and many other problems. A plant-based diet can help in maintaining healthy cholesterol levels.

- **Ramping Up Your Plant Intake May Keep Your Brain Strong**
  Increased consumption of fruits and vegetables is associated with a 20 percent reduction in the risk of cognitive impairment and dementia. So plant foods can help protect your brain from multiple issues.

What to Eat in Plant-Based Diets

Fruits: Berries, citrus fruits, pears, peaches, pineapple, bananas, etc.

Vegetables: Kale, spinach, tomatoes, broccoli, cauliflower, carrots, asparagus, peppers, etc.

Starchy vegetables: Potatoes, sweet potatoes, butternut squash, etc.

Whole grains: Brown rice, rolled oats, farro, quinoa, brown rice pasta, barley, etc.

Healthy fats: Avocados, olive oil, coconut oil, unsweetened coconut, etc.

Legumes: Peas, chickpeas, lentils, peanuts, black beans, etc.

Seeds, nuts, and nut butters: Almonds, cashews, macadamia nuts, pumpkin seeds, sunflower seeds, natural peanut butter, tahini, etc.

Unsweetened plant-based milks: Coconut milk, almond milk, cashew milk, etc.

Spices, herbs, and seasonings: Basil, rosemary, turmeric, curry, black pepper, salt, etc.

Condiments: Salsa, mustard, nutritional yeast, soy sauce, vinegar, lemon juice, etc.

Plant-based protein: Tofu, tempeh, plant-based protein sources or powders with no added sugar or artificial ingredients.

Beverages: Coffee, tea, sparkling water, etc.

What Not to Eat in Plant-Based Diets

Fast food: French fries, cheeseburgers, hot dogs, chicken nuggets, etc.

Added sugars and sweets: Table sugar, soda, juice, pastries, cookies, candy, sweet tea, sugary cereals, etc.

Refined grains: White rice, white pasta, white bread, bagels, etc.

Packaged and convenience foods: Chips, crackers, cereal bars, frozen dinners, etc.

Processed vegan-friendly foods: Plant-based meats like; Tofurkey, faux cheeses, vegan butters, etc.

Artificial sweeteners: Equal, Splenda, Sweet'N Low, etc.

Processed animal products: Bacon, lunch meats, sausage, beef jerky, etc.

Day 1:

Breakfast (304 calories)

- 1 serving Berry-Kefir Smoothie

A.M. Snack (95 calories)

- 1 medium apple

Lunch (374 calories)

- 1 serving Green Salad with Pita Bread & Hummus

P.M. Snack (206 calories)

- 1/4 cup dry-roasted unsalted almonds

Dinner (509 calories)

- 1 serving Beefless Vegan Tacos
- 2 cups mixed greens
- 1 serving Citrus Vinaigrette

Day 2:

Breakfast (258 calories)

- 1 serving Cinnamon Roll Overnight Oats
- 1 medium orange

A.M. Snack (341 calories)

- 1 cup low-fat plain Greek yogurt
- 1 medium peach
- 3 tbsps slivered almonds

Lunch (332 calories)

- 1 serving Thai-Style Chopped Salad with Sriracha Tofu

P.M. Snack (131 calories)

- 1 large pear

Dinner (458 calories)

- 1 serving Mexican Quinoa Salad

Day 3:

Breakfast (258 calories)

- 1 serving Cinnamon Roll Overnight Oats
- 1 medium orange

A.M. Snack (95 calories)

- 1 medium apple

Lunch (463 calories)

- 1 serving Thai-Style Chopped Salad with Sriracha Tofu
- 1 large pear

P.M. Snack (274 calories)

- 1/3 cup dried walnut halves
- 1 medium peach

Dinner (419 calories)

- 1 serving Eggs in Tomato Sauce with Chickpeas & Spinach
- 1 1-oz. slice whole-wheat baguette

BREAKFAST

Almond Granola with Resins

Servings: 4

Preparation Time: 20 minutes

Per Serving:

Ingredients:

- 1/8 tsp ground allspice
- 1/4 cup shelled sunflower seeds
- 1/2 cup golden raisins
- 1/2 cup shaved almonds
- 3 cups old-fashioned oats
- 3/4 cups chopped walnuts
- 1/2 tsp ground cinnamon
- 1/2 cup pure maple syrup
- A pinch of salt

Procedure:

1. First, preheat the oven to 325 F.
2. In a baking dish, place the oats, walnuts, and sunflower seeds. Bake for 10 minutes.
3. Then lower the heat from the oven to 300 F.
4. Stir in the raisins, almonds, maple syrup, cinnamon, allspice, and salt.
5. Now bake for an additional 15 minutes.
6. Allow cooling before serving.

Pecan & Pumpkin Seed Oat Jars

Servings: 10

Preparation Time: 10 minutes

Ingredients:

- 5 cups old-fashioned rolled oats
- 5 tsps agave syrup
- Salt to taste
- 2 tsps ground cardamom
- 10 tbsps pumpkin seeds
- 10 tbsps chopped pecans
- 10 cups unsweetened soy milk
- 2 tsps ground ginger

Procedure:

1. Take a bowl, put oats, pumpkin seeds, pecans, soy milk, agave syrup, salt, cardamom, and ginger and toss to combine.
2. Then divide the mixture between mason jars.
3. Finally, seal the lids and transfer them to the fridge to soak for 10-12 hours.

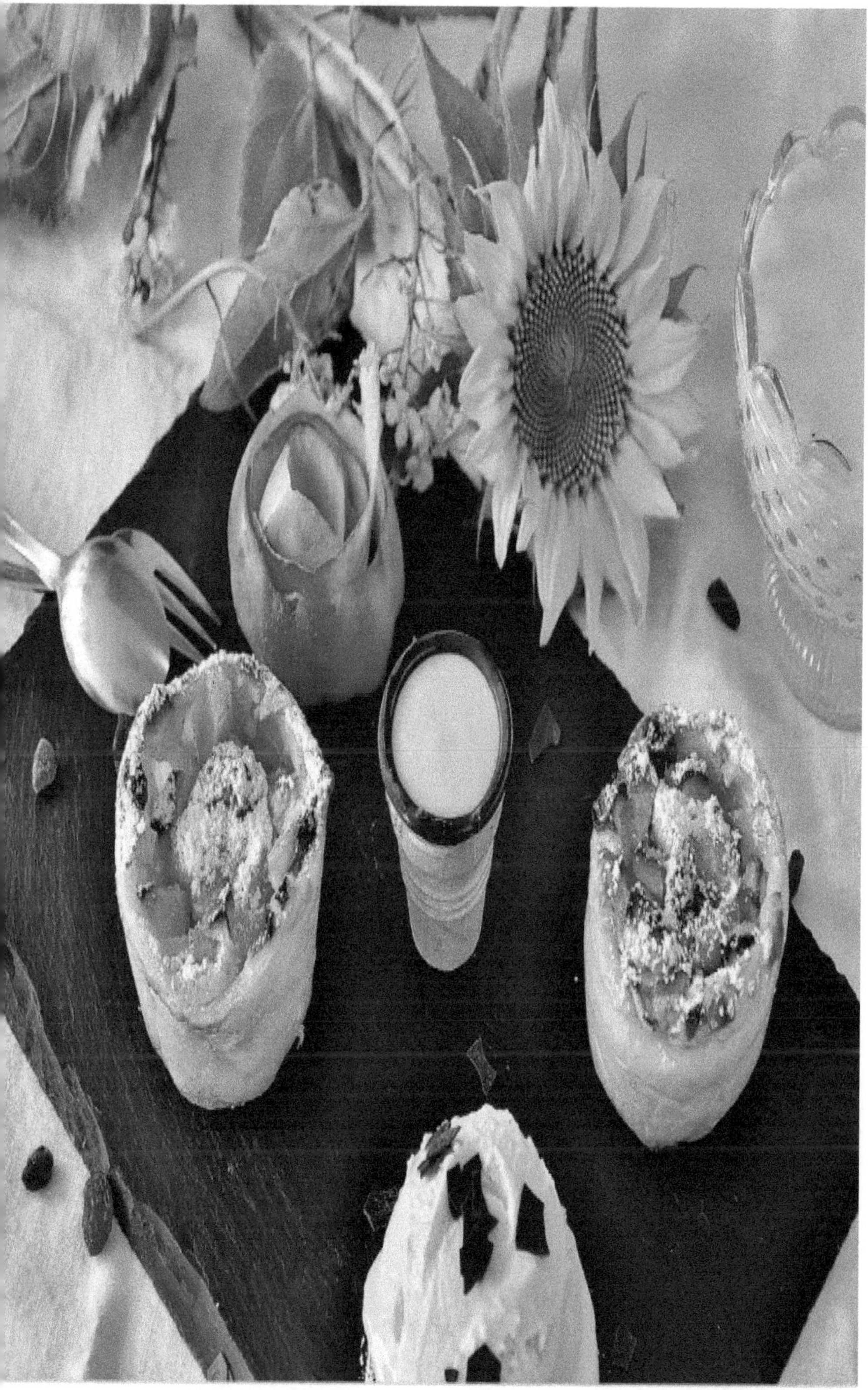

Apple Muffins

Servings: 8

Preparation Time: 40 minutes

Ingredients:

For the muffins:

- 1/4 cup melted plant butter
- 14 cup flax milk
- 4 apples, chopped
- 1 1/2 cup pure date sugar
- 4 tsps baking powder
- 2 flax seeds powder
- 6 tbsps water
- 3 cups whole-wheat flour
- 2 tsps cinnamon powder
- 1/2 tsp salt

For topping:

- 1 cup pure date sugar
- 1 cup cold plant butter, cubed
- ½ cup whole-wheat flour
- 3 tsp cinnamon powder

Procedure:

1. First of all, preheat the oven to 400 F and grease 6 muffin cups with cooking spray.

2. Then take a bowl, mix the flax seed powder with water and allow thickening for 5 minutes to make the vegan "flax egg."
   Take a bowl, mix flour, date sugar, baking powder, salt, and cinnamon powder.
3. Whisk in the butter, vegan "flax egg," flax milk, and fold in the apples.
4. Fill the muffin cups two-thirds way up with the batter.
5. Take a bowl, mix the remaining flour, date sugar, cold butter, and cinnamon powder.
6. Now sprinkle the mixture on the muffin batter.
7. Finally, bake for 20 minutes. Remove the muffins onto a wire rack, allow cooling, and serve.

Easy Avocado Toast with Herbs & Peas

Servings: 8

Preparation Time: 10 minutes

Per Serving: Calories: 250 Cal Fat: 12 g Carbs: 22 g Protein: 7 g Fiber: 9 g

Ingredients:

- 1 of a medium avocado, peeled, pitted, mashed
- 2 teaspoons chopped basil
- ½ teaspoon salt
- 12 slices of radish
- 1/2 teaspoon ground black pepper
- 1 lemon, juiced
- 2 slices of bread, whole-grain, toasted
- 4 tablespoons baby peas

Procedure:

1. First of all, spread mashed avocado on one side of the toast and then top with peas, pressing them into the avocado.
2. Then layer the toast with radish slices, season with salt and black pepper, sprinkle with basil, and drizzle with lemon juice.
3. Finally, serve straight away.

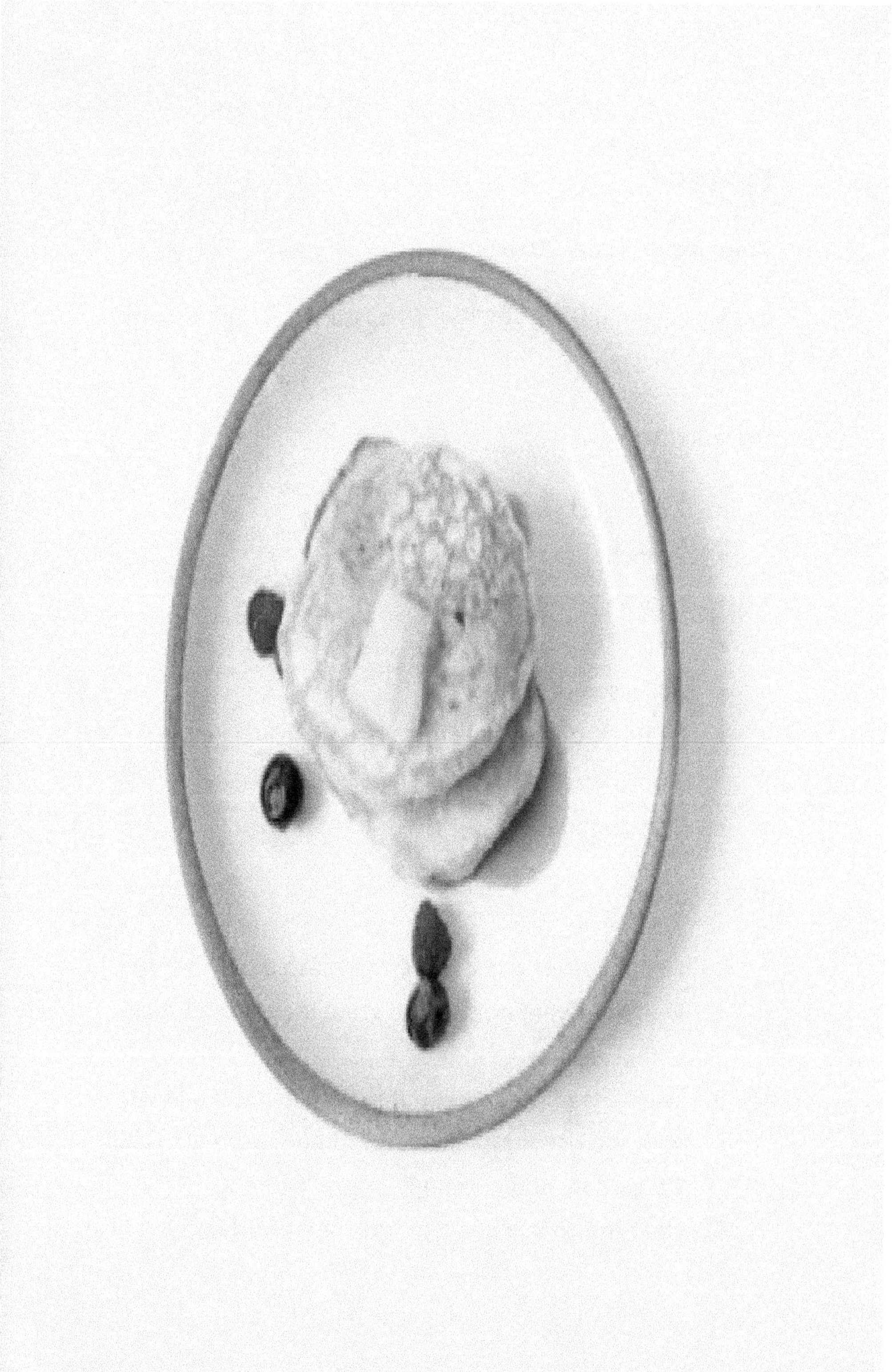

Small Sized Sweet Potato Pancakes

Servings: 4

Preparation Time: 20 minutes

Per Serving: Calories: 209 Fat: 15.4g Carbs: 10.5g Protein: 8.1g Fiber: 3.2g

Ingredients:

- 2 cloves of garlic
- 2 pinches of nutmeg
- 6 tablespoons of water
- Salt
- 300 g sweet potato
- 6 tablespoons whole meal rice flour
- 2 pinches of chili flakes
- 2 teaspoons oil

Procedure:

1. First, peel the garlic clove and mash it with a fork.
2. Peel the sweet potato and grate it into small sticks with a greater.
3. Then knead the sweet potato and garlic in a bowl with the rice flour and water, then season with chili flakes, salt, and nutmeg.
4. Heat the oil in a pan and form small buffers.

5. Now fry these in the pan on both sides until golden brown.
6. Goes perfectly with tzatziki and other fresh dips.

Sprout Toast with Avocado

Servings: 8

Preparation Time: 5 minutes

Per Serving: Calories: 200 Cal Fat: 10.5 g Carbs: 22 g
Protein: 7 g Fiber: 7 g

Ingredients:

- 1 of a medium avocado, sliced
- 1/2 teaspoon lemon zest
- 1 teaspoon hemp seeds
- 1/2 teaspoon red pepper flakes
- 2 slices of whole-grain bread, toasted
- 4 tablespoons sprouts
- 4 tablespoons hummus

Procedure:

1. First, spread hummus on one side of the toast and then top with avocado slices and sprouts.
2. Now sprinkle with lemon zest, hemp seeds, and red pepper flakes, and then serve straight away.

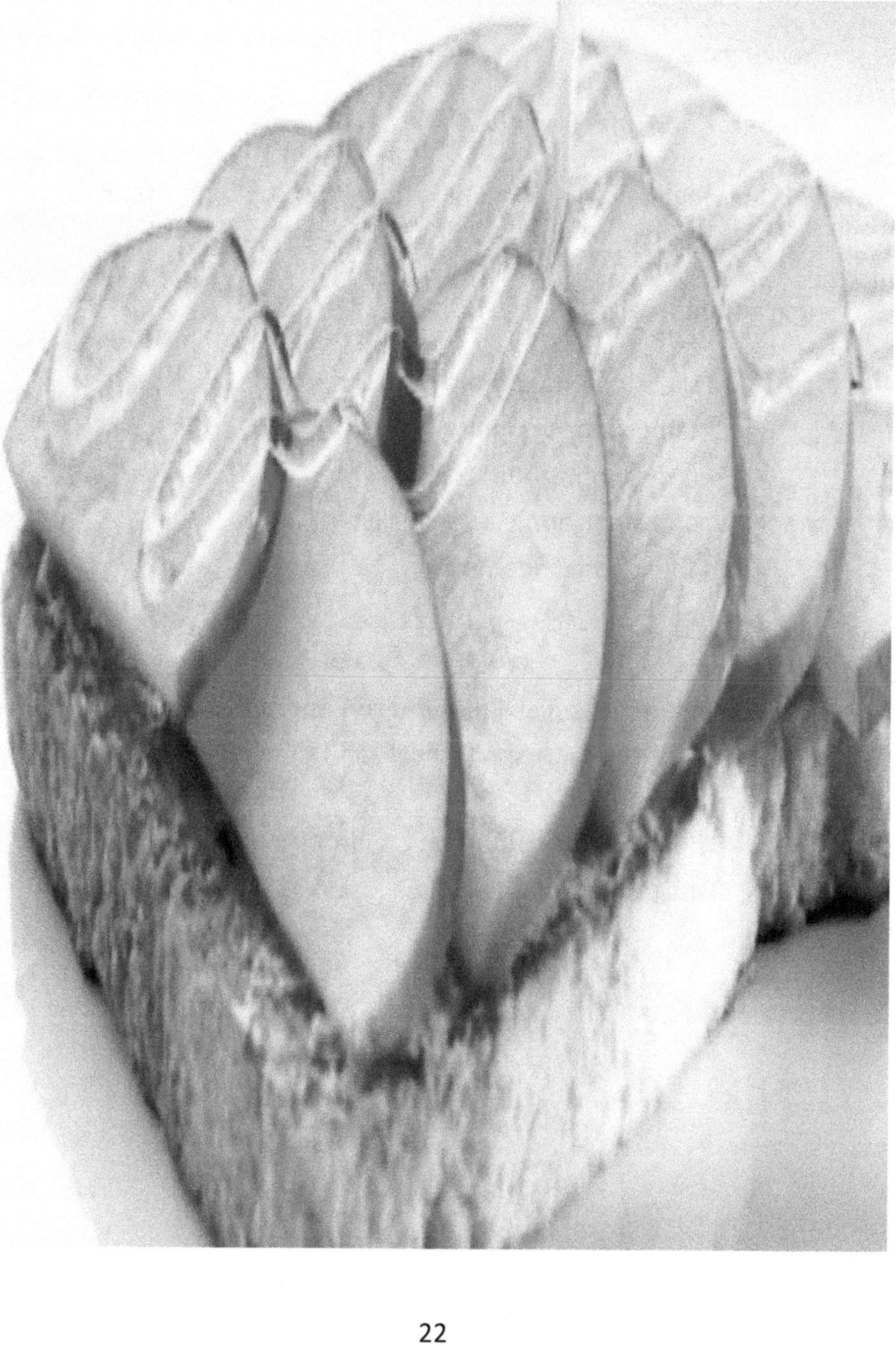

Honey Apple Toast

Servings: 8

Preparation Time: 5 minutes

Per Serving: Calories: 212 Cal Fat: 7 g Carbs: 35 g Protein: 4 g Fiber: 5.5 g

Ingredients:

- 2 slices of whole-grain bread, toasted
- 2 tablespoons honey
- 4 tablespoons hummus
- 1 of a small apple, cored, sliced
- ¼ teaspoon cinnamon

Procedure:

1. First of all, spread hummus on one side of the toast, top with apple slices, and then drizzle with honey.
2. Then sprinkle cinnamon on it and then serve straight away.

Morning Cinnamon Semolina Porridge

Servings: 6

Preparation Time: 20 minutes

Per Serving: Calories: 491; Fat: 13.2g; Carbs: 76g; Protein: 16.6g

Ingredients:

- 6 cups almond milk
- 1/2 teaspoon kosher salt
- 1 teaspoon ground cinnamon
- 6 tablespoons maple syrup
- 6 teaspoons coconut oil
- 2 1/2 cups semolina

Procedure:

1. Take a saucepan, heat the almond milk, maple syrup, coconut oil, salt, and cinnamon over a moderate flame.
2. Once hot, gradually stir in the semolina flour.
3. Then turn the heat to a simmer and continue cooking until the porridge reaches your preferred consistency.
4. Finally, garnish with your favorite toppings and serve warm.

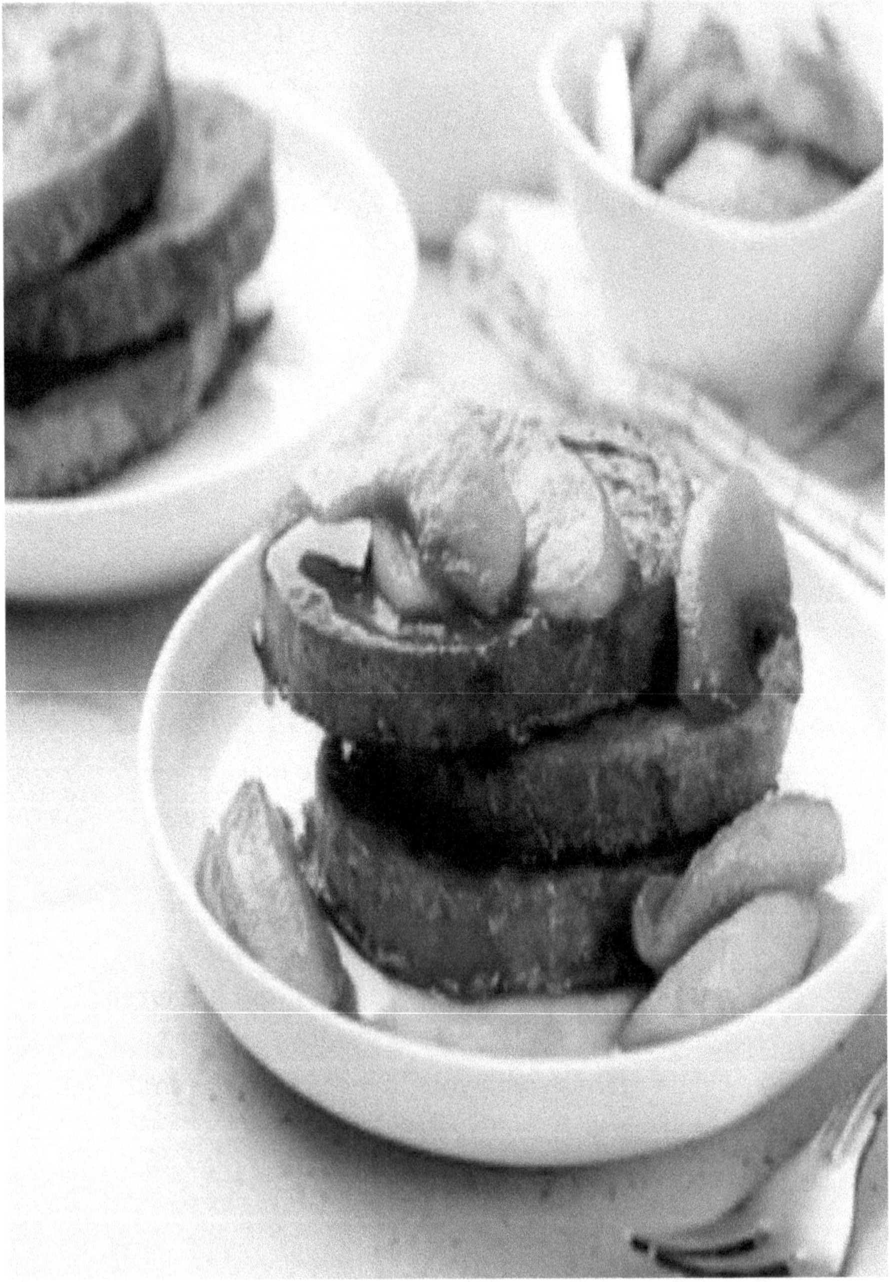

Apple sauce French Toast

Servings: 2

Preparation Time: 15 minutes

Per Serving: Calories: 333; Fat: 16.9g; Carbs: 40.3g; Protein: 5.6g

Ingredients:

- 2 pinches of grated nutmeg
- 1/2 teaspoon ground cloves
- 1/2 teaspoon ground cinnamon
- 4 slices rustic day-old bread slices
- 2 tablespoons coconut oil
- 2 tablespoons maple syrup
- 1/2 cup oat milk, sweetened
- 4 tablespoons applesauce, sweetened
- 1 teaspoon vanilla paste
- 2 pinches of salt

Procedure:

1. Take a mixing bowl, thoroughly combine the oat milk, applesauce, vanilla, salt, nutmeg, cloves, and cinnamon.
2. Dip each slice of bread into the custard mixture until well coated on all sides.
3. Then preheat the coconut oil in a frying pan over medium-high heat. Cook for about 3 minutes on each side until golden brown.
4. Now drizzle the French toast with maple syrup and serve immediately.

Morning Bread Pudding with Nuts

Servings: 12

Preparation Time: 2 hours 10 minutes

Per Serving: Calories: 463; Fat: 6.2g; Carbs: 83g; Protein: 11.4g

Ingredients:

- 3 cups almond milk
- 1 cup maple syrup
- 1 teaspoon ground cloves
- 1/4 teaspoon kosher salt
- 1 teaspoon ground cinnamon
- 8 cups day-old white bread, cubed
- 1 cup almonds, roughly chopped
- 4 tablespoons almond butter
- 1 teaspoon vanilla extract
- 1 teaspoon almond extract

Procedure:

1. Take a mixing bowl, combine the almond milk, maple syrup, almond butter, vanilla extract, almond extract, and spices.
2. Then add the bread cubes to the custard mixture and stir to combine well. Fold in the almonds and allow it to rest for about 1 hour.
3. Then, spoon the mixture into a lightly oiled casserole dish.

4. Now bake in the preheated oven at 350 degrees F for about 1 hour or until the top is golden brown.
5. Place the bread pudding on a wire rack for 10 minutes before slicing and serving.

Frosty Blackberry Smoothie with Hemp

Servings: 4

Preparation Time: 10 minutes

Per Serving: Calories: 362; Fat: 9.1g; Carbs: 52.1g; Protein: 22.1g

Ingredients:

- 2 cups coconut yogurt
- 2 cups blackberries, frozen
- 4 small-sized bananas, frozen
- 2 tablespoons hemp seeds
- 1 cup coconut milk
- 8 tablespoons granola

Procedure:

1. Take your blender, mix all ingredients, trying to keep the liquids at the bottom of the blender to help it break up the fruits.
2. Then divide your smoothie between serving bowls.
3. Garnish each bowl with granola and some extra frozen berries, if desired.
   Finally, serve immediately!

Steel Cut Chocolate & Walnut Oats

Servings: 6

Preparation Time: 30 minutes

Per Serving: Calories: 452; Fat: 18.1g; Carbs: 67g; Protein: 11g

Ingredients:

- 4 cups oat milk
- ½ teaspoon cinnamon powder
- ½ teaspoon vanilla extract
- 8 tablespoons cocoa powder
- 1/4 cup steel-cut oats
- 2 tablespoons coconut oil
- ½ cup coconut sugar
- 2 pinches of grated nutmeg
- 2 pinches of flaky sea salt
- 1/4 cup English walnut halves
- 8 tablespoons chocolate chips

Procedure:

1. First, bring the oat milk and oats to a boil over moderately high heat.
2. Then, turn the heat to low and add in the coconut oil, sugar, and spices; let it simmer for about 25 minutes, stirring periodically.

3. Now add in the cocoa powder and continue simmering for an additional 3 minutes.
4. Spoon the oatmeal into serving bowls.
5. Finally, top each bowl with the walnut halves and chocolate chips.

LUNCH

Easy Carrot & Mushroom Broth

Servings: 12

Preparation Time: 1 hour 15 minutes

Ingredients:

- 1 cup chopped fresh parsley
- Salt and black pepper to taste
- 2 medium carrots, coarsely chopped
- 2 celery ribs with leaves, chopped
- 10 dried porcini mushrooms, soaked and liquid reserved
- 2 tbsps olive oil
- 2 onions, unpeeled and quartered
- 2 onions, chopped
- 16 oz. Cremini mushrooms, chopped
- 10 cups water

Procedure:

1. First, warm the oil in a pot over medium heat.
2. Place in onion, carrot, celery, and cremini mushrooms.
3. Cook for 5 minutes until softened. Add in the dried mushrooms and reserved liquid, onion, salt, and water. Bring to a boil and simmer for 1 hour.

4. Let cool for a few minutes, and then pour over a strainer into a pot. Divide between glass mason jars and allow cooling completely.
5. Finally, seal and store in the fridge for up to 5 days or 1 month in the freezer.

Corn & Fennel Chowder

Servings: 8

Preparation Time: 30 minutes

Per Serving:

Ingredients:

- 4 tbsps olive oil
- 2 onions, chopped
- 4 cups canned corn
- 4 cups cubed red potatoes
- 1/2 cup whole-wheat flour
- 8 cups vegetable stock
- 1 tsp chili paste
- Sea salt and black pepper to taste
- 2 cups almond milk
- 2 cups chopped fennel bulb
- 4 carrots, chopped
- 2 cups mushrooms, chopped

Procedure:

1. First, heat the oil in a pot over medium heat.
2. Then place in onion, fennel, carrots, and mushrooms.
3. Sauté for 5 minutes until tender.
4. Stir in flour and pour in vegetable stock.

5. Now lower the heat and add in corn, potatoes, almond milk, and chili paste.
6. Simmer for 20 minutes and sprinkle with salt and pepper.
7. Finally, serve immediately.

Parsnip Bisque with Fennel

Servings: 12

Preparation Time: 30 minutes

Ingredients:

- 1/2 tsp dried marjoram
- 12 cups vegetable broth
- 2 cups plain unsweetened soy milk
- 4 parsnips, shredded
- 2 potatoes, chopped
- 4 garlic cloves, minced
- 2 tbsps olive oil
- 4 green onions, chopped
- 1 fennel bulb, sliced
- 4 large carrots, shredded
- 2 tsps dried thyme
- 2 tbsps minced fresh parsley

Procedure:

1. First, heat the oil in a pot over medium heat.
2. Place in green onions, fennel, carrots, parsnips, potato, and garlic.
3. Then sauté for 5 minutes until softened.
4. Add in thyme, marjoram, and broth. Bring to a boil, lower the heat, and simmer for 20 minutes.

5. Now transfer to a blender and pulse the soup until smooth. Return to the pot and mix in soy milk.
6. Top with parsley to serve.

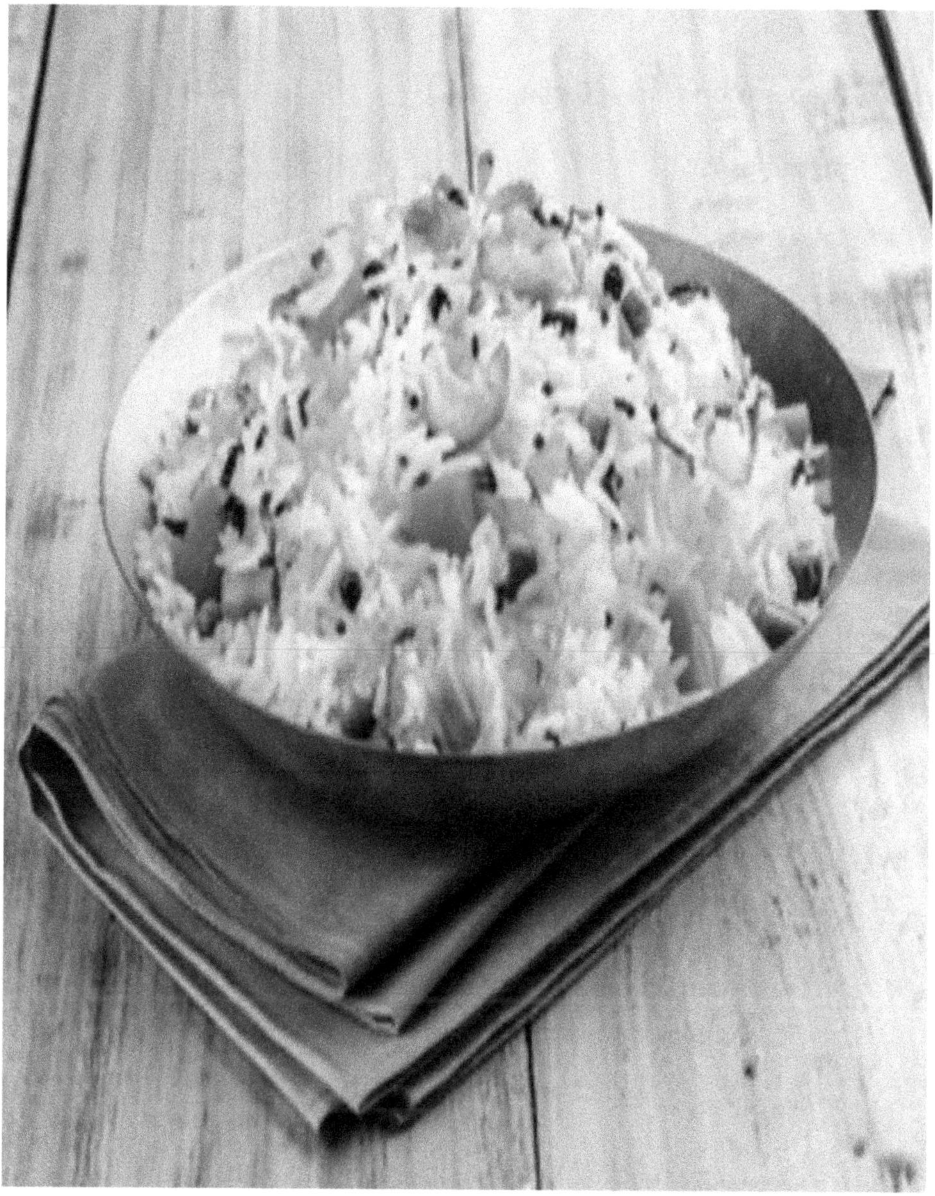

Easy Mushroom & Green Bean Biryani

Servings: 8

Preparation Time: 50 minutes

Ingredients:

- 4 tsps garam masala
- 2 tbsps tomato puree
- 2 cups chopped cremini mushrooms
- 2 cups brown rice
- 6 tbsps plant butter
- 6 medium white onions, chopped
- 12 garlic cloves, minced
- 1 tsp cardamom powder
- 1 tsp cayenne powder
- 2 tsps ginger puree
- 2 tbsps turmeric powder + for dusting
- 1/2 tsp cinnamon powder
- 1 tsp cumin powder
- 2 tsps smoked paprika
- 6 large tomatoes, diced
- 4 green chilies, minced
- 2 cups chopped mustard greens
- 2 cups plant-based yogurt

Procedure:

1. First, melt the butter in a large pot and sauté the onions until softened, 3 minutes.

2. Mix in the garlic, ginger, turmeric, cardamom powder, garam masala, cardamom powder, cayenne pepper, cumin powder, paprika, and salt.
3. Then stir-fry for 1-2 minutes.
4. Stir in the tomatoes, green chili, tomato puree, and mushrooms.
5. Once boiling, mix in the rice and cover it with water.
6. Now cover the pot and cook over medium heat until the liquid absorbs and the rice is tender for 15-20 minutes.
7. Open the lid and fluff in the mustard greens and half of the parsley.
8. Finally, dish the food, top with the coconut yogurt, garnish with the remaining parsley and serve warm.

Homemade Baked Cheese Spaghetti Squash

Servings: 8

Preparation Time: 40 minutes

Ingredients:

Baked Cheesy Spaghetti Squash

Ingredients for 4 servings

- 1/3 tsp chili powder
- 2 cups coconut cream
- 4 oz. cashew cream cheese
- 2 tbsps coconut oil
- Salt and black pepper to taste
- 4 tbsps melted plant butter
- 1 tbsp garlic powder
- 4 oz. grated plant-based Parmesan
- 4 tbsps fresh cilantro, chopped
- Olive oil for drizzling
- 2 cups plant-based mozzarella
- 4 lbs spaghetti squash

Procedure:

1. First, preheat the oven to 350 F.
2. Cut the squash in halves lengthwise and spoon out the seeds and fiber.
3. Then place on a baking dish, brush with coconut oil, and season with salt and pepper.

4. Now bake for 30 minutes.
5. Remove and use two forks to shred the flesh into strands.
6. After that, empty the spaghetti strands into a bowl and mix with plant butter, garlic and chili powders, coconut cream, cream cheese, half of the plant-based mozzarella, and plant-based Parmesan cheeses.
7. Spoon the mixture into the squash cups and sprinkle with the remaining mozzarella cheese.
8. Finally, bake further for 5 minutes. Sprinkle with cilantro and drizzle with some oil, and serve.

Easy Mongolian Seitan

Servings: 8

Preparation Time: 50 minutes

Per Serving: Calories 354 kcal Fats 20. 8g Carbs 17.7g
Protein 25.2g

Ingredients:

For the sauce:

- 1 cup low-sodium soy sauce
- 1 cup + 4 tbsps pure date sugar
- 4 tsps cornstarch
- 4 tbsps cold water
- 4 tsps olive oil
- 1 tsp freshly grated ginger
- 6 garlic cloves, minced
- 1/2 tsp red chili flakes
- 1/2 tsp allspice

For the crisped seitan:

- 2 lbs. seitan, cut into 1-inch pieces
- 3 tbsps olive oil

For topping:

- 2 tbsps sliced scallions
- 2 tbsps toasted sesame seeds

Procedure:

1. First, heat the olive oil in a wok and sauté the ginger and garlic until fragrant, 30 seconds.
2. After that, mix in the red chili flakes, Chinese allspice, soy sauce, and date sugar.
3. Then allow the sugar to melt and set aside.
4. Take a small bowl, mix the cornstarch and water.
5. Stir the cornstarch mixture into the sauce and allow thickening for 1 minute. Turn the heat off.
6. Now heat the olive oil in a medium skillet over medium heat and fry the seitan on both sides until crispy, 10 minutes,
7. Mix the seitan into the sauce and warm over low heat.
8. Dish the food, garnish with sesame seeds and scallions.
9. Serve warm with brown rice.

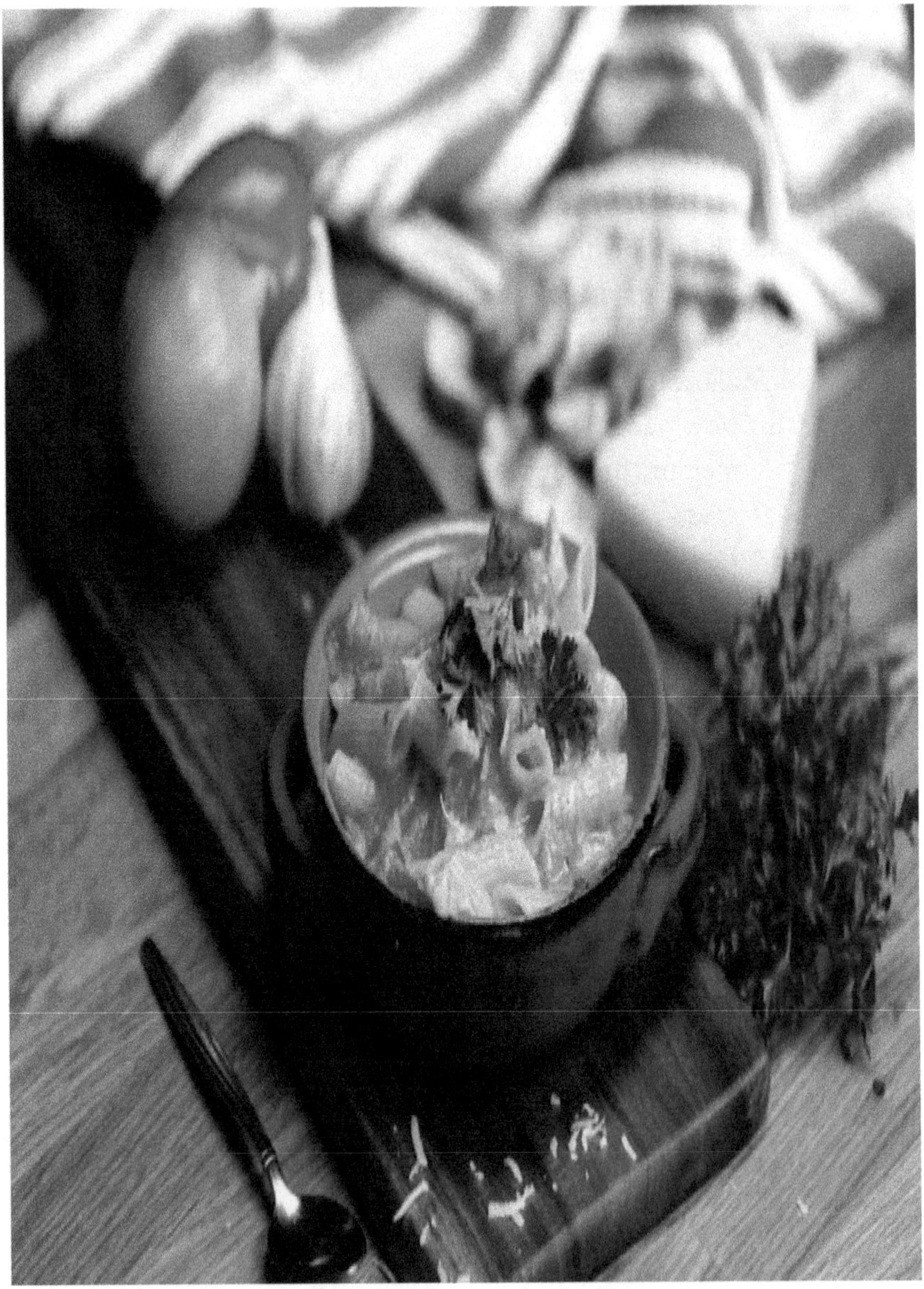

Cherry Tomato Alfredo Pasta

Servings: 8

Preparation Time: 50 minutes

Per Serving: Calories 698 kcal Fats 26.1g Carbs 101.8g
Protein 22.6g

Ingredients:

- 32 oz. whole-wheat fettuccine
- 1 cup coconut cream
- 6 tbsps plant butter
- 2 large garlic cloves, minced
- Salt and black pepper to taste
- Chopped fresh parsley to garnish
- 1/2 cup halved cherry tomatoes
- 1 1/2 cups grated plant-based Parmesan cheese
- 4 cups almond milk
- 3 cups vegetable broth

Procedure:

1. First, bring almond milk, vegetable broth, butter, and garlic to a boil in a large pot, 5 minutes.
2. Mix in the fettuccine and cook until tender while frequently tossing around 10 minutes.

3. Then mix in coconut cream, tomatoes, plant Parmesan cheese, salt, and pepper.
4. Now cook for 3 minutes or until the cheese melts.
5. Garnish with some parsley and serve warm.

Chard Wraps with Millet

Servings: 8

Preparation Time: 25 minutes

Per Serving: Calories: 152 Cal Fat: 4. 5 g Carbs: 25 g
Protein: 3. 5 g Fiber: 2. 4 g

Ingredients:

- 1 of a large cucumber cut into ribbons
- 1 cup chickpeas, cooked
- 2 cups sliced cabbage
- 2 carrots cut into ribbons
- 1 cup millet, cooked
- 1/2 cup hummus

Topping:

- Mint Leaves
- Hemp seeds
- 2 bunches of Swiss rainbow chard

Procedure:

1. First of all, spread hummus on one side of the
   chard, place some millet, vegetables, and chickpeas
   on it, sprinkle with some mint leaves and hemp
   seeds and wrap it like a burrito.
2. Then serve straight away.

Special Quinoa Meatballs

Servings: 8

Preparation Time: 10 minutes

Per Serving: Calories: 100 Cal Fat: 100 g Carbs: 100 g Protein: 100 g Fiber: 100 g

Ingredients:

- 2 cups quinoa, cooked
- 2 cups grated vegan mozzarella cheese
- 2 tablespoons flax meal
- 2 cups diced white onion
- 2 teaspoons paprika
- 2 teaspoons dried basil
- 6 tablespoons water
- 4 tablespoons olive oil
- 3 teaspoons minced garlic
- 1 teaspoon salt
- 2 teaspoons dried oregano
- 2 teaspoons lemon zest
- Marinara sauce as needed for serving

Procedure:

1. First, place flax meal in a bowl, stir in water, and set aside until required.
2. Take a large skillet pan, place it over medium heat, add 1 tablespoon oil and when hot, add onion and cook for 2 minutes.
3. Then stir in all the spices and herbs and then stir in quinoa until combined and cook for 2 minutes.

4. Now transfer quinoa mixture in a bowl, add flax meal mixture, lemon zest, and cheese, stir until well mixed and then shape the mixture into twelve 1 ½ inch balls.
5. After that, arrange balls on a baking sheet lined with parchment paper, refrigerate the balls for 30 minutes and then bake for 20 minutes at 400 degrees F.
6. Serve balls with marinara sauce.

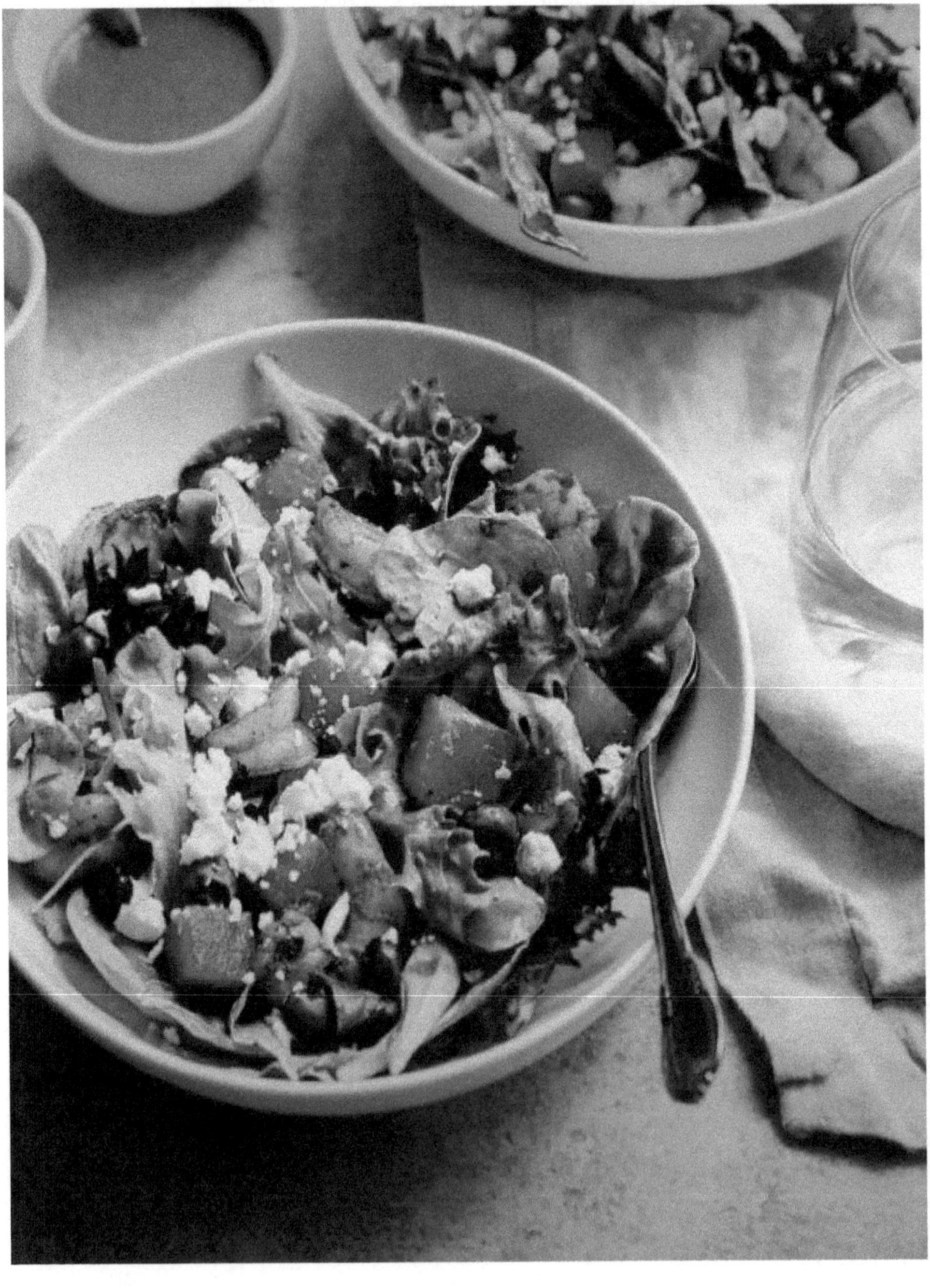

Herbs Beluga Lentil Salad

Servings: 8

Preparation Time: 20 minutes

Per Serving: Calories: 364; Fat: 17g; Carbs: 40.2g; Protein: 13.3g

Ingredients:

- 2 green bell peppers, seeded and diced
- 2 red bell peppers, seeded and diced
- 1 teaspoon garlic, minced
- 2 teaspoons agave syrup
- 4 tablespoons fresh lemon juice
- 2 teaspoons lemon zest
- 4 tablespoons fresh parsley, roughly chopped
- 2 cups red lentils
- 6 cups water
- 2 cups grape tomatoes, halved
- 4 tablespoons fresh cilantro, roughly chopped
- 4 tablespoons fresh chives, roughly chopped
- 4 tablespoons fresh basil, roughly chopped
- 1/2 cup olive oil
- 1 teaspoon cumin seeds
- 1 teaspoon ginger, minced
- Sea salt and ground black pepper, to taste
- 4 ounces black olives, pitted and halved
- 2 red chili peppers, seeded and diced
- 2 cucumbers, sliced

- 8 tablespoons shallots, chopped

Procedure:

1. First of all, add the brown lentils and water to a saucepan and bring to a boil over high heat.
2. Then, turn the heat to a simmer and continue to cook for 20 minutes or until tender.
3. Now place the lentils in a salad bowl.
4. Add in the vegetables and herbs and toss to combine well.
5. Take a mixing bowl; whisk the oil, cumin seeds, ginger, garlic, agave syrup, lemon juice, lemon zest, salt and black pepper.
6. In conclusion, dress your salad, garnish with olives and serve at room temperature.

Italian-Style Bean Salad

Servings: 8

Preparation Time: 1 hour

Per Serving: Calories: 495; Fat: 21.1g; Carbs: 58.4g; Protein: 22.1g

Ingredients:

- 2 tablespoons lime juice
- 2 teaspoon Italian herb mix
- Kosher salt and ground black pepper, to season
- 2 red onions, thinly sliced
- 2 teaspoon garlic, minced
- 1 1/2 pound cannellini beans, soaked overnight and drained
- 4 cups cauliflower florets
- 1/2 cup extra-virgin olive oil
- 1 teaspoon ginger, minced
- 2 teaspoon Dijon mustard
- 1/2 cup white vinegar
- 4 cloves garlic, pressed
- 2 jalapeno peppers, minced
- 2 cups grape tomatoes, quartered
- 4 ounces green olives, pitted and sliced

Procedure:

1. First cover the soaked beans with a fresh change of cold water and bring to a boil.
2. Let it boil for about 10 minutes.

3. Then turn the heat to a simmer and continue to cook for 60 minutes or until tender.
4. Meanwhile, boil the cauliflower florets for about 6 minutes or until just tender.
5. Now allow your beans and cauliflower to cool completely; then, transfer them to a salad bowl.
6. Then add in the remaining ingredients and toss to combine well.
7. Taste and adjust the seasonings.

Coconut Sorghum Porridge

Servings: 4

Preparation Time: 15 minutes

Per Serving: Calories: 289; Fat: 5.1g; Carbs: 57.8g; Protein: 7.3g

Ingredients:

- 1/2 teaspoon grated nutmeg
- 1 cup sorghum
- 1/2 teaspoon ground cloves
- 1 teaspoon ground cinnamon
- Kosher salt, to taste
- 4 tablespoons agave syrup
- 2 cups water
- 1 cup coconut milk
- 4 tablespoons coconut flakes

Procedure:

1. First, place the sorghum, water, milk, nutmeg, cloves, cinnamon, and kosher salt in a saucepan; simmer gently for about 15 minutes.
2. Spoon the porridge into serving bowls.
3. In conclusion, top with agave syrup and coconut flakes.

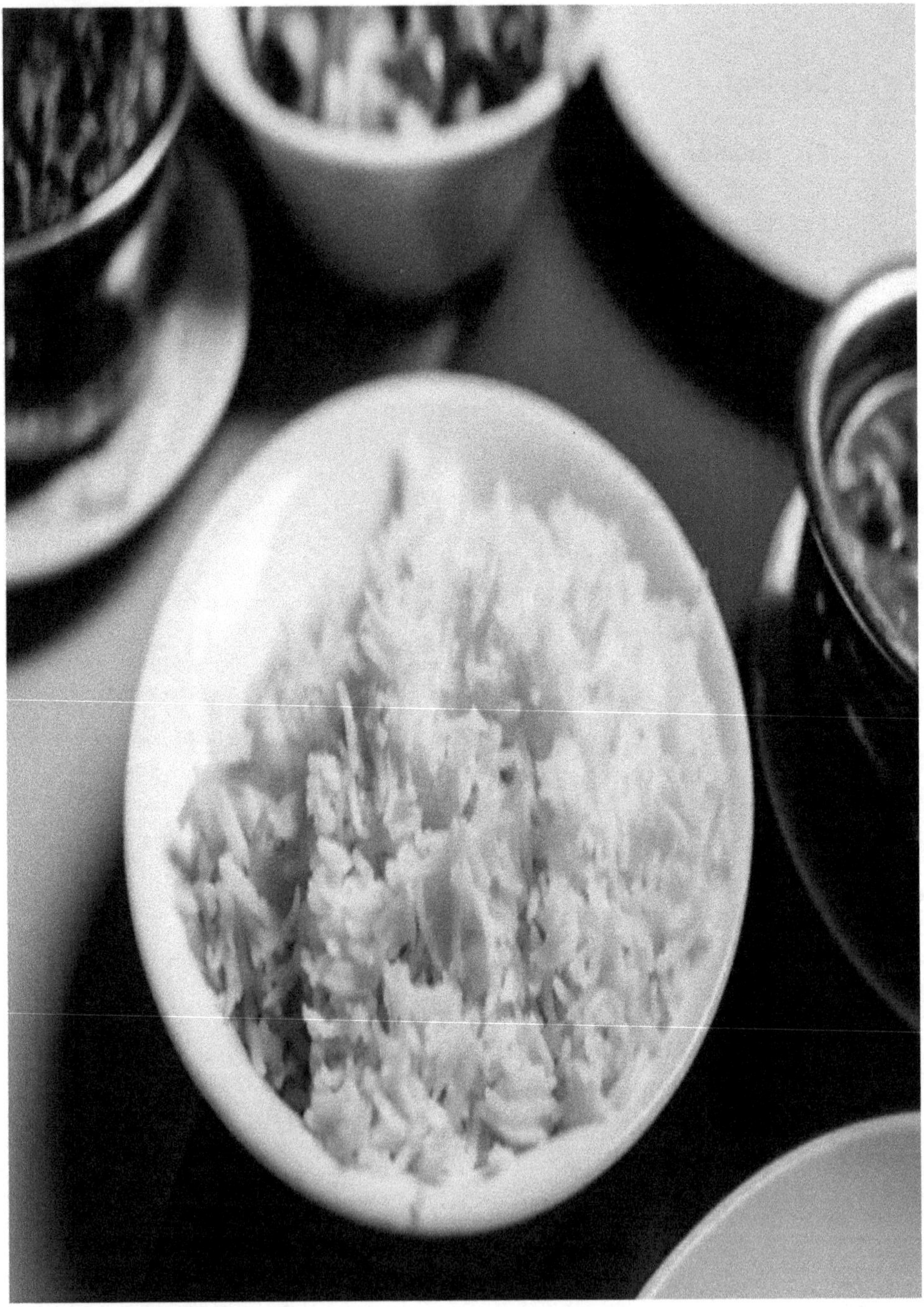

Aromatic Rice

Servings: 8

Preparation Time: 20 minutes

Per Serving: Calories: 384; Fat: 11.4g; Carbs: 60.4g; Protein: 8.3g

Ingredients:

- 6 tablespoons olive oil
- 2 bays leaves
- 2 teaspoons dried oregano
- 3 cups white rice
- 5 cups vegetable broth
- Sea salt and cayenne pepper, to taste
- 2 teaspoons garlic, minced
- 2 teaspoons dried rosemary

Procedure:

1. Take a saucepan, heat the olive oil over a moderately high flame.
2. Add in the garlic, oregano, rosemary, and bay leaf; sauté for about 1 minute or until aromatic.
3. Add in the rice and broth.
4. Bring to a boil; immediately turn the heat to a gentle simmer.

5. Cook for about 15 minutes or until all the liquid has been absorbed.
6. Fluff the rice with a fork, season with salt and pepper, and serve immediately.

DINNER

Easy Cherry & Pistachio Bulgur

Servings: 8

Preparation Time: 45 minutes

Ingredients:

- 1 cup chopped pistachios
- 2 carrots, chopped
- 2 celery stalks, chopped
- 2 tbsps plant butter
- 2 white onions, chopped
- 8 cups vegetable broth
- 2 cups chopped dried cherries, soaked
- 2 cups chopped mushrooms
- 3 cups bulgur

Procedure:

1. First, preheat the oven to 375 F.
2. Melt butter in a skillet over medium heat.
3. Sauté the onion, carrot, and celery for 5 minutes until tender.
4. Then add in mushrooms and cook for 3 more minutes.
5. Pour in bulgur and broth.

6. Now transfer to a casserole and bake covered for 30 minutes.
7. Once ready, uncover and stir in cherries.
8. Top with pistachios to serve.

Bean & Brown Rice with Artichokes

Servings: 8

Preparation Time: 35 minutes

Ingredients:

- 4 tbsps olive oil
- 6 garlic cloves, minced
- 2 cups artichokes hearts, chopped
- 2 tsps dried basil
- 3 cups cooked navy beans
- 3 cups long-grain brown rice
- 2 cups vegetable broth
- Salt and black pepper to taste
- 4 ripe grape tomatoes, quartered
- 4 tbsps minced fresh parsley

Procedure:

1. First of all, heat the oil in a pot over medium heat.
2. Sauté the garlic for 1 minute.
3. Then stir in artichokes, basil, navy beans, rice, and broth.
4. Sprinkle with salt and pepper.
5. Now lower the heat and simmer for 20-25 minutes.
6. Remove to a bowl and mix in tomatoes and parsley.
7. Using a fork, fluff the rice and serve right away.

Homemade Pressure Cooker Celery & Spinach Chickpeas

Servings: 10

Preparation Time: 50 minutes

Ingredients:

- 4 garlic cloves, minced
- 2 tbsps coconut oil
- 2 cups chickpeas, soaked overnight
- 2 celery stalks, chopped
- 4 tbsps olive oil
- 6 tsps ground cinnamon
- 1 tsp ground nutmeg
- 2 onions, chopped
- 3 cups spinach, chopped

Procedure:

1. Firstly, place chickpeas in your IP with the onion, garlic, celery, olive oil, 2 cups of water, cinnamon, and nutmeg.
2. Then lock the lid in place; set the time to 30 minutes on High.
3. Once ready, perform a natural pressure release for 10 minutes.
4. Now unlock the lid and drain the excess water.

5. Put back the chickpeas and stir in coconut oil and spinach.
6. Finally, set the pot to Sauté and cook for another 5 minutes.

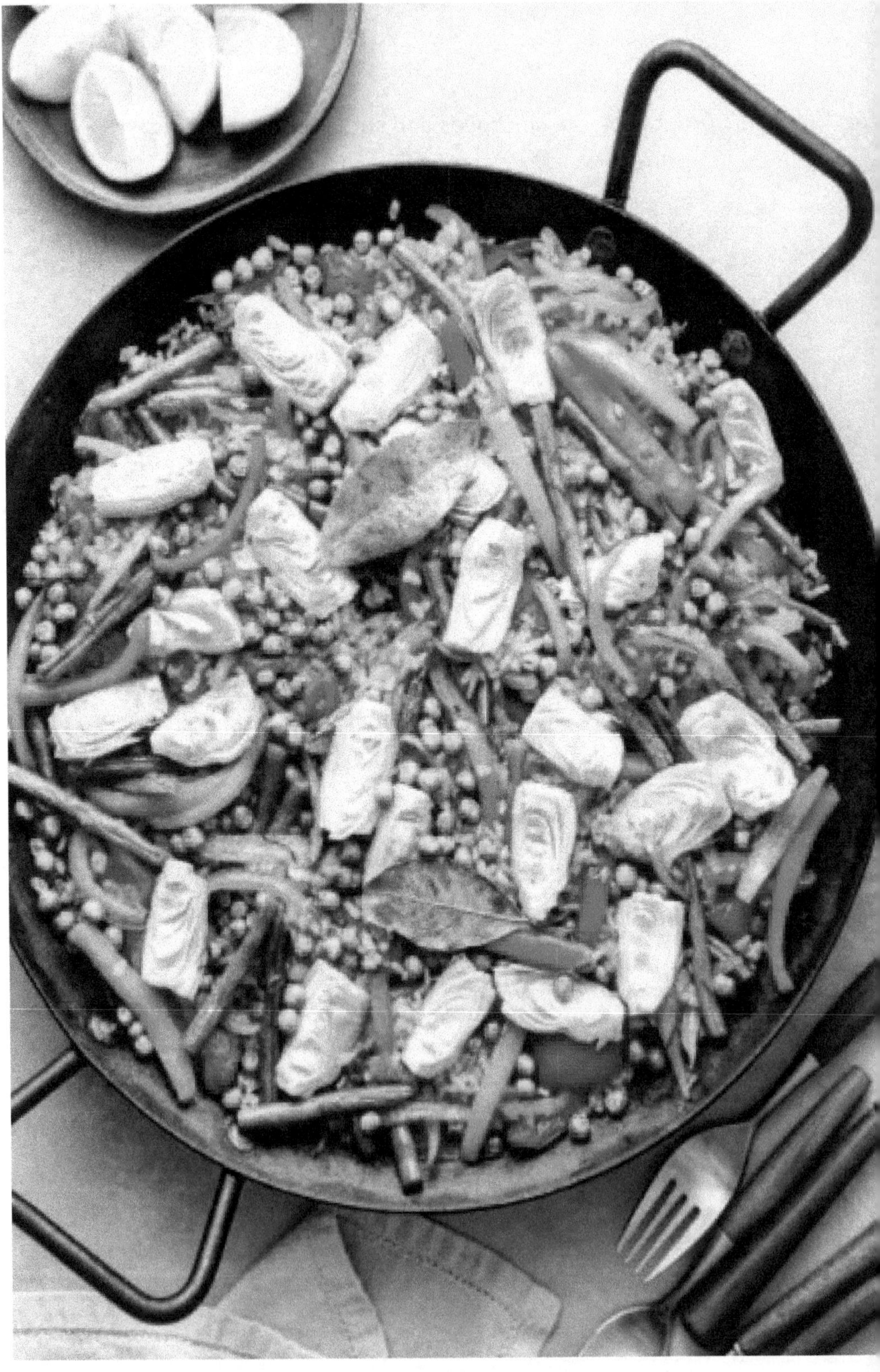

Easy Vegetable Paella with Lentils

Servings: 8

Preparation Time: 50 minutes

Ingredients:

- 4 tbsps olive oil
- 2 onions, chopped
- 3 cups long-grain brown rice
- 6 cups vegetable broth
- 2 tbsps capers
- 1/2 tsp crushed red pepper
- 1/2 cup sliced pitted black olives
- 4 tbsps minced fresh parsley
- 3 cups cooked lentils, drained
- 2 green bell peppers, chopped
- 4 garlic cloves, minced
- 2 (29-oz) cans diced tomatoes

Procedure:

1. Initially, heat oil in a pot over medium heat and sauté onion, bell pepper, and garlic for 5 minutes.
2. Then stir in tomatoes, capers, red pepper, and salt. Cook for 5 minutes. Pour in the rice and broth.
3. Bring to a boil, and then lower the heat.

4. Now simmer for 20 minutes.
5. Turn the heat off and mix in lentils.
6. In the end, serve garnished with olives and parsley.

Amazing Curry Beans with Artichokes

Servings: 8

Preparation Time: 25 minutes

Ingredients:

- 2 tsps olive oil
- 2 small onions, diced
- 4 tsps curry powder
- 1 tsp ground coriander
- 2 (10.5-oz) cans coconut milk
- 4 garlic cloves, minced
- 2 (29-oz) cans cannellini beans
- 2 (29-oz) cans artichoke hearts, drained and quartered
- Salt and black pepper to taste

Procedure:

1. Initially, heat the oil in a skillet over medium heat.
2. Sauté the onion and garlic for 3 minutes until translucent.
3. Then stir in beans, artichoke, curry powder, and coriander.
4. Add in coconut milk.
5. Now bring to a boil, then lower the heat and simmer for 10 minutes. Serve.

Creamy Peas Fettuccine

Servings: 8

Preparation Time: 40 minutes

Per Serving: Calories 654 Fats 23.7g Carbs 101.9g Protein 18.2g

Ingredients:

- 1 cup cashew butter, room temperature
- 32 oz. whole-wheat fettuccine
- Salt and black pepper to taste
- 2 tbsps olive oil
- 4 garlic cloves, minced
- 3 cups frozen peas
- 1 1/2 cup flax milk
- 1 cup chopped fresh basil

Procedure:

1. First, add the fettuccine and 10 cups of water to a large pot, and cook over medium heat until al dente, 10 minutes.
2. Drain the pasta through a colander and set it aside.
3. Take a bowl, whisk the flax milk, cashew butter, and salt until smooth and set aside.
4. Then, heat the olive oil in a large skillet and sauté the garlic until fragrant, 30 seconds.

5. Mix in the peas, fettuccine, and basil.
6. Now toss well until the pasta is well-coated in the sauce and season with some black pepper.
7. In conclusion, dish the food and serve warm.

Easy Buckwheat Cabbage Rolls

Servings: 8

Preparation Time: 30 minutes

Per Serving: Calories 1147 Fats 112.9g Carbs 25.6g Protein 23.8g

Ingredients:

- 1 medium sweet onion, finely chopped
- 4 tbsps plant butter
- 4 cups extra-firm tofu, pressed and crumbled
- 4 garlic cloves, minced
- 2 bays leafs
- 4 tbsps chopped fresh cilantro + more for garnishing
- 2 head Savoy cabbages, leaves separated (scraps kept)
- 2 (46 oz.) canned chopped tomatoes
- Salt and black pepper to taste
- 2 cups buckwheat groats
- 3 1/2 cups vegetable stock

Directions:

1. First, melt the plant butter in a large bowl and cook the tofu until golden brown, 8 minutes.
2. Stir in the onion and garlic until softened and fragrant, 3 minutes.

3. Season with salt, black pepper, and mix in the buckwheat, bay leaf, and vegetable stock.
4. Then close the lid, allow boiling, and then simmer until all the liquid is absorbed.
5. Open the lid; remove the bay leaf, adjust the taste with salt, black pepper, and mix in the cilantro.
6. Now lay the cabbage leaves on a flat surface and add 3 to 4 tablespoons of the cooked buckwheat onto each leaf.
7. Roll the leaves to firmly secure the filling.
8. After that, pour the tomatoes with juices into a medium pot, season with a little salt, black pepper, and lay the cabbage rolls in the sauce.
9. Then cook over medium heat until the cabbage softens, 5 to 8 minutes.
10. Turn the heat off and dish the food onto serving plates.
11. Finally, garnish with more cilantro and serve warm.

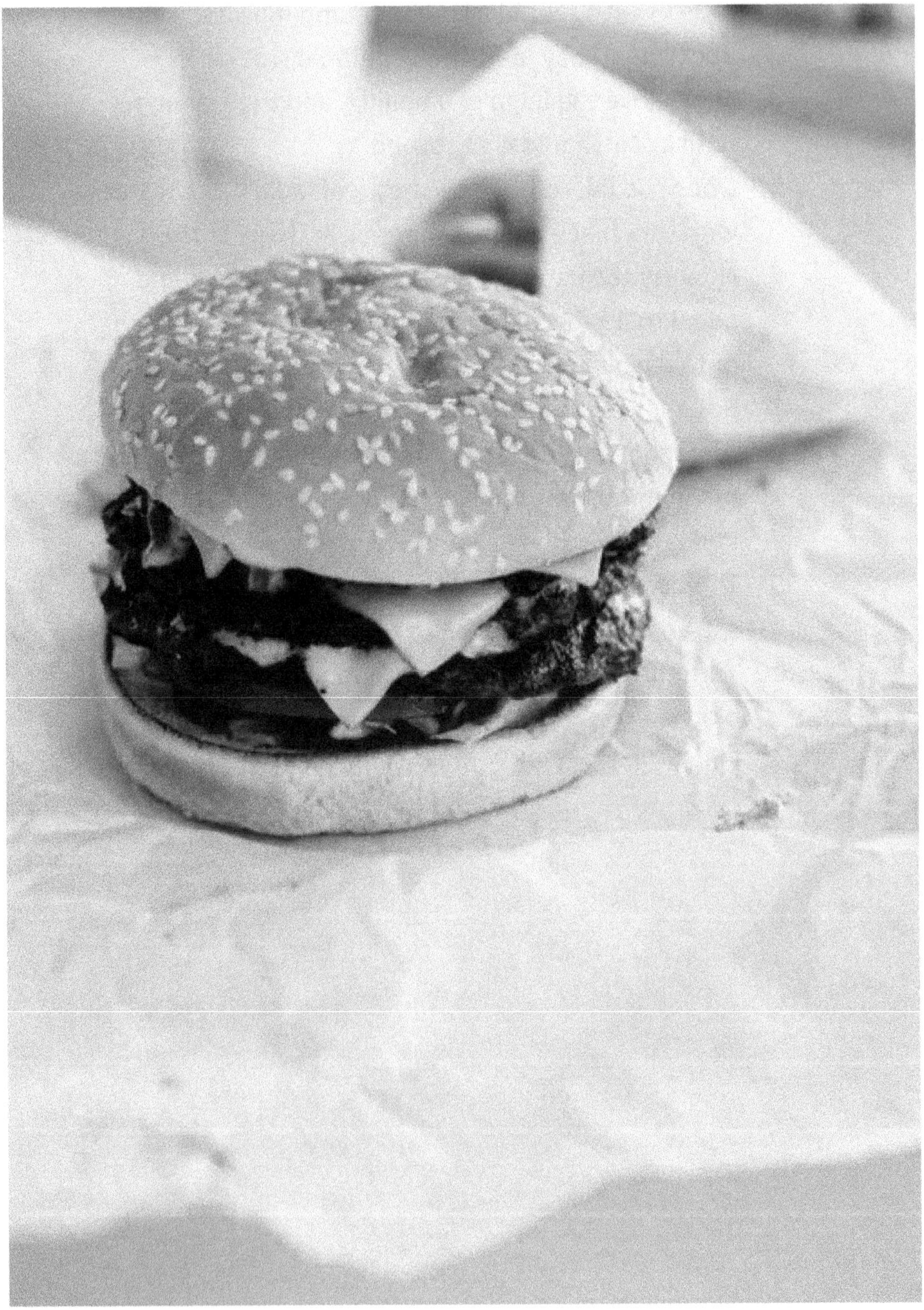

Black Beans BBQ Burgers

Servings: 8

Preparation Time: 15-30 minutes

Per Serving: Calories 589 Fats 17.7g Carbs 80.9g Protein 27.9g

Ingredients:

- 4 tbsps pure barbecue sauce
- 2 garlic cloves, minced
- Salt and black pepper to taste
- 6 (30 oz.) cans black beans, drained and rinsed
- 4 tbsps whole-wheat flour
- 4 tbsps quick-cooking oats
- 1/2 cup chopped fresh basil
- 8 whole-grain hamburger buns split

For topping:

- Red onion slices
- Fresh basil leaves
- Additional barbecue sauce
- Tomato slices

Directions:

1. First, take a medium bowl, mash the black beans and mix in the flour, oats, basil, barbecue sauce, garlic salt, and black pepper until well combined.

2. Then mold 4 patties out of the mixture and set them aside.
3. Heat a grill pan to medium heat and lightly grease with cooking spray.
4. Now cook the bean patties on both sides until light brown and cooked through, 10 minutes.
5. After that, place the patties between the burger buns and top with the onions, tomatoes, basil, and some barbecue sauce.
6. Serve warm.

Tomato & Paprika Pasta Primavera

Servings: 8

Preparation Time: 15-30 minutes

Per Serving: Calories 380 kcal Fats 24.1g Carbs 33.7g
Protein 11.2g

Ingredients:

- 2 small red onions, sliced
- 4 garlic cloves, minced
- 2 cups dry white wine
- 4 tbsps olive oil
- 16 oz. whole-wheat fedelini
- Salt and black pepper to taste
- 4 cups cherry tomatoes, halved
- 6 tbsps plant butter, cut into ½-in cubes
- 1 tsp paprika
- 2 lemons, zested and juiced
- 2 cups packed fresh basil leaves

Procedure:

1. First of all, heat the olive oil in a large pot and mix
   in the fedelini, paprika, onion, garlic, and stir-fry for
   2-3 minutes.
2. Mix in the white wine, salt, and black pepper.
3. Then cover with water.

4. Cook until the water absorbs and the fedelini al dente, 5 minutes.
5. After that, mix in the cherry tomatoes, plant butter, lemon zest, lemon juice, and basil leaves.
6. In conclusion, dish the food and serve warm.

Green Lentils Stew & Brown Rice

Servings: 8

Preparation Time: 15-30 minutes

Ingredients:

For the stew:

- 2 tsps chili powder
- 2 tsps onion powder
- 4 tbsps olive oil
- 2 lb. tempeh, cut into cubes
- Salt and black pepper to taste
- 2 tsps cumin powder
- 4 celeries stalks, chopped
- 4 cups vegetable broth
- 2 tsps oregano
- 2 cups green lentils, rinsed
- 1/2 cup chopped tomatoes
- 2 limes, juiced
- 4 carrots diced
- 8 garlic cloves, minced
- 2 tsps garlic powder
- 2 yellow onions, chopped

For the brown rice:

- 2 cups of water
- 2 cups of brown rice
- Salt to taste

Procedure:

1. First, heat the olive oil in a large pot, season the tempeh with salt, black pepper, and cook in the oil until brown, 10 minutes.
2. Then stir in the chili powder, onion powder, cumin powder, garlic powder, and cook until fragrant, 1 minute.
3. Mix in the onion, celery, carrots, garlic, and cook until softened.
4. Now pour in the vegetable broth, oregano, green lentils, tomatoes, and green chilies.
5. Cover the pot and cook until the tomatoes soften and the stew reduces by half, 10 to 15 minutes.
6. After that, open the lid, adjust the taste with salt, black pepper, and mix in the lime juice.
7. Dish the stew and serve warm with the brown rice.
8. Meanwhile, as the stew cooks, add the brown rice, water, and salt to a medium pot.
9. Finally, cook over medium heat until the rice is tender and the water is absorbed for about 15 to 25 minutes.

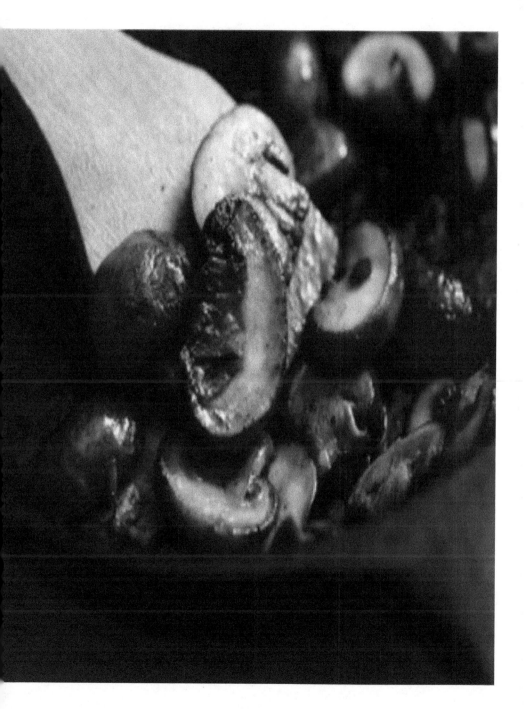

Herb Garlic Mushroom Skillet

Servings: 8

Preparation Time: 10 minutes

Per Serving: Calories: 207; Fat: 15.2g; Carbs: 12.7g; Protein: 9.1g

Ingredients:

- 3 pounds oyster mushrooms halved
- 8 tablespoons vegan butter
- 2 teaspoons dried parsley flakes
- 2 teaspoons dried marjoram
- 1 cup dry white wine
- Kosher salt and ground black pepper, to taste
- 6 cloves of garlic, minced
- 2 teaspoons dried oregano
- 2 teaspoons dried rosemary

Procedure:

1. Take a sauté pan, heat the olive oil over moderately high heat.
2. Now, sauté the mushrooms for 3 minutes or until they release the liquid.
3. Then add in the garlic and continue to cook for 30 seconds more or until aromatic.
4. Stir in the spices and continue sautéing for an additional 6 minutes until your mushrooms are lightly browned.

Fried Asparagus

Servings: 8

Preparation Time: 10 minutes

Per Serving: Calories: 142; Fat: 11.8g; Carbs: 7.7g; Protein: 5.1g

Ingredients:

- 1/2 teaspoon bay leaf, ground
- Sea salt and ground black pepper, to taste
- 2 teaspoons fresh lime juice
- 8 tablespoons vegan butter
- 3 pounds asparagus spears, trimmed
- 1 teaspoon cumin seeds, ground

Procedure:

1. First, melt the vegan butter in a saucepan over medium-high heat.
2. Sauté the asparagus for about 3 to 4 minutes, stirring periodically to promote even cooking.
3. Then add in the cumin seeds, bay leaf, salt, and black pepper and continue to cook the asparagus for 2 minutes more until crisp-tender.
4. Now drizzle lime juice over the asparagus and serve warm.

Ginger Carrot Mash

Servings: 8

Preparation Time: 25 minutes

Per Serving: Calories: 187; Fat: 8.4g; Carbs: 27.1g; Protein: 3.4g

Ingredients:

- 4 pounds carrots cut into rounds
- 1 teaspoon cayenne pepper
- 1 teaspoon ginger, peeled and minced
- 4 tablespoons olive oil
- 2 teaspoons ground cumin
- Salt ground black pepper, to taste
- 1 cup whole milk

Procedure:

1. First, begin by preheating your oven to 400 degrees F.
2. Toss the carrots with olive oil, cumin, salt, black pepper, and cayenne pepper. Arrange them in a single layer on a parchment-lined roasting sheet.
3. Then roast the carrots in the preheated oven for about 20 minutes, until crisp-tender.
4. Now add the roasted carrots, ginger, and milk to your food processor; puree the ingredients until everything is well blended.

DRINKS

Energizing Cinnamon Detox Tonic

Servings: 4

Preparation Time: 40 minutes

Per Serving: Calories:80 Cal, Carbohydrates:0g, Protein:0g, Fats:0g, Fiber:0g.

Ingredients:

- 2 teaspoons of maple syrup
- 2 teaspoons of apple cider vinegar
- 1/4 teaspoon of cayenne pepper
- 1/4 teaspoon of ground turmeric
- 4 cups of boiling water
- 8 sticks of cinnamon 2 inches each
- 2 small lemon slices

Procedure:

1. First, pour the boiling water into a small saucepan, add and stir the cinnamon sticks, then let it rest for 8 to 10 minutes before covering the pan.
2. Pass the mixture through a strainer and into the liquid; add the cayenne pepper, turmeric, cinnamon, and stir properly.
3. Then add the maple syrup, vinegar, and lemon slice.
4. Finally, add and stir an infused lemon and serve immediately.

Cherry Cinnamon Cider

Servings: 8

Preparation Time: 5 hours

Per Serving: Calories:100 Cal, Carbohydrates:0g, Protein:0g, Fats:0g, Fiber:0g.

Ingredients:

- 3-ounce of cherry gelatin
- 2 quarts of apple cider
- 1 cinnamon sticks, each about 3 inches long

Procedure:

1. Using a 6-quart slow cooker, pour the apple cider and add the cinnamon stick.
2. Then stir, then cover the slow cooker with its lid. Plug the cooker and let it cook for 3 hours at the high heat setting or until it is heated thoroughly.
3. Then add and stir the gelatin properly, then continue cooking for another hour.
4. When done, remove the cinnamon sticks and serve the drink hot or cold.

Warm Pomegranate Punch

Servings: 10

Preparation Time: 2 hours

Per Serving: Calories: 253 Cal, Carbohydrates: 58g, Protein: 7g, Fats: 2g, Fiber: 3g.

Ingredients:

- 1/3 cup of lemon juice
- 32 fluid ounce of pomegranate juice
- 32 fluid ounce of apple juice, unsweetened
- 3 cinnamon sticks, each about 3 inches long
- 12 whole cloves
- 1/2 cup of coconut sugar
- 16 fluid ounce of brewed tea

Procedure:

1. Using a 4-quart slow cooker, pour the lemon juice, pomegranate juice, apple juice, tea, and then sugar.
2. Then wrap the whole cloves and cinnamon stick in cheesecloth, tie its corners with a string, and immerse it in the liquid present in the slow cooker.
3. Then cover it with the lid, plug in the slow cooker and let it cook at the low heat setting for 3 hours or until it is heated thoroughly.
4. When done, discard the cheesecloth bag and serve it hot or cold.

Truffle Hot Chocolate

Servings: 8

Preparation Time: 1.5 hour

Per Serving: Calories: 67 Cal, Carbohydrates: 13g, Protein: 2g, Fats: 2g, Fiber: 2.3g.

Ingredients:

- 1/4 teaspoon of ground cinnamon
- 2 teaspoons of vanilla extract, unsweetened
- 64 fluid ounce of coconut milk
- 1/4 teaspoon of salt
- 1/2 cup of cocoa powder, unsweetened
- 1/2 cup of coconut sugar

Procedure:

1. Using a 2 quarts slow cooker, add all the ingredients, and stir properly.
2. Then cover it with the lid, then plug in the slow cooker and cook it for 2 hours on the high heat setting or until it is heated thoroughly.
3. Finally, serve right away.

Spiced Warm lemon Drink

Servings: 12

Preparation Time: 2 hours

Per Serving: Calories: 15 Cal, Carbohydrates:3. 2g, Protein:0. 1g, Fats: 0g, Fiber:0g.

Ingredients:

- 2 cinnamon sticks, about 3 inches long
- 1 teaspoon of whole cloves
- 24 fluid ounce of orange juice
- 5 quarts of water
- 8 fluid of ounce pineapple juice
- 1 cup and 4 tablespoons of lemon juice
- 4 cups of coconut sugar

Procedure:

1. First of all, pour water into a 6-quart slow cooker and stir the sugar and lemon juice properly.
2. Wrap the cinnamon, the whole cloves in cheesecloth, and tie its corners with string.
3. Then immerse this cheesecloth bag in the liquid present in the slow cooker and cover it with the lid.
4. Then plug in the slow cooker and let it cook on a high heat setting for 2 hours or until it is heated thoroughly.
5. Now discard the cheesecloth bag and serve the drink hot or cold.

Mulled Wine

Servings: 12

Preparation Time: 40 minutes

Per Serving: Calories: 202 Cal, Carbohydrates:25g, Protein:0g, Fats:0g, Fiber:0g.

Ingredients:

- 2 tablespoons of star anise
- ½ cup of honey
- 16 fluid ounce of apple cider
- 48 fluid ounce of red wine
- 16 fluid ounce of cranberry juice
- 2 cups of cranberries, fresh
- 4 oranges, juiced
- 2 tablespoons of whole cloves
- 4 cinnamon sticks, each about 3 inches long

Procedure:

1. Using a 4 quarts slow cooker, add all the ingredients, and stir properly.
2. Then cover it with the lid, then plug in the slow cooker and cook it for 30 minutes on the high heat setting or until it gets warm thoroughly.
3. Finally, strain the wine and serve right away.

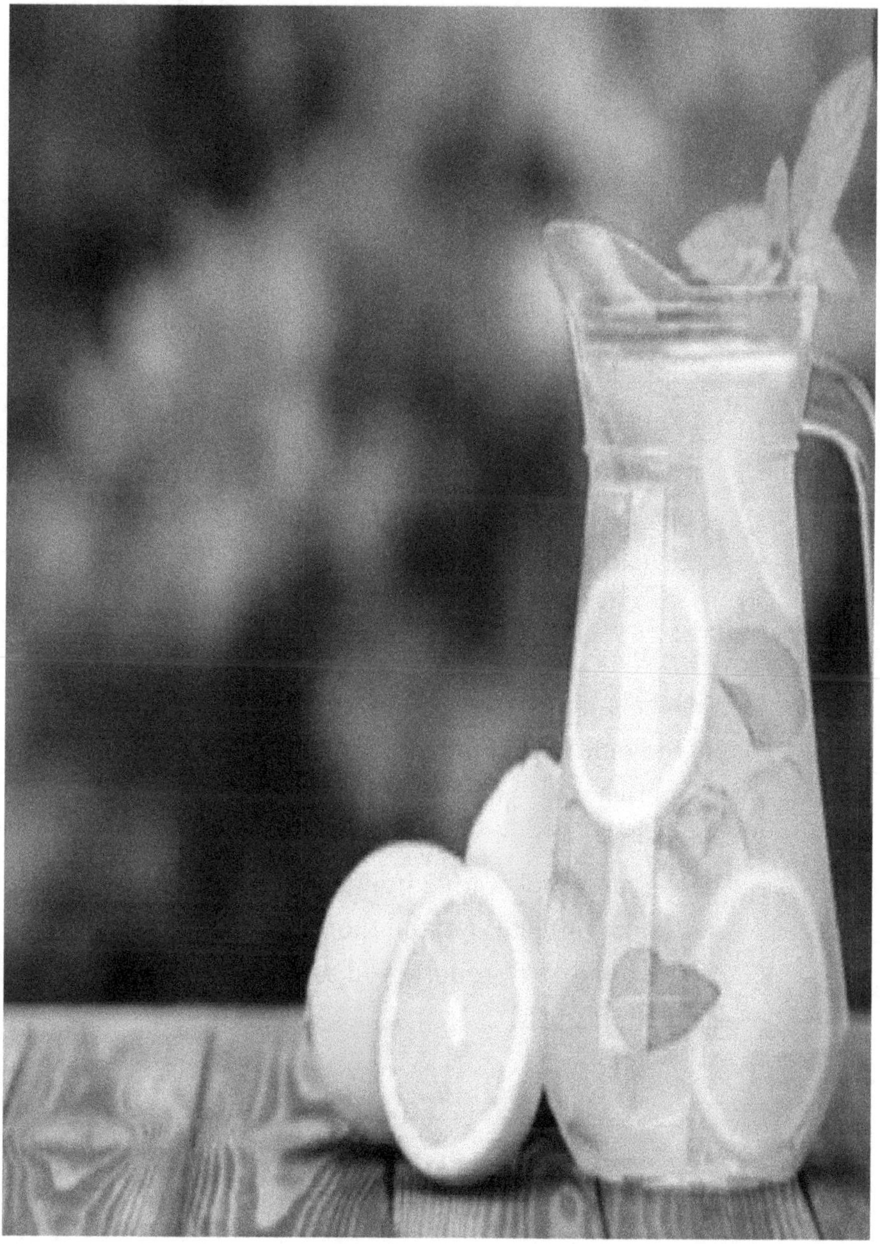

Pleasant Homemade Lemonade

Servings: 10

Preparation Time: 15 minutes

Per Serving: Calories: 146 Cal, Carbohydrates: 34g, Protein:0g, Fats:0g, Fiber:0g.

Ingredients:

- 6 cups of lemon juice fresh
- 64 fluid ounce of water
- Cinnamon sticks for serving
- 4cups of coconut sugar
- 1/2 cup of honey

Procedure:

1. Using a 4-quart slow cooker, place all the ingredients except for the cinnamon sticks and stir properly.
2. Then cover it with the lid, then plug in the slow cooker and cook it for 3 hours on the low heat setting or until it is heated thoroughly.
3. When done, stir properly and serve with the cinnamon sticks.

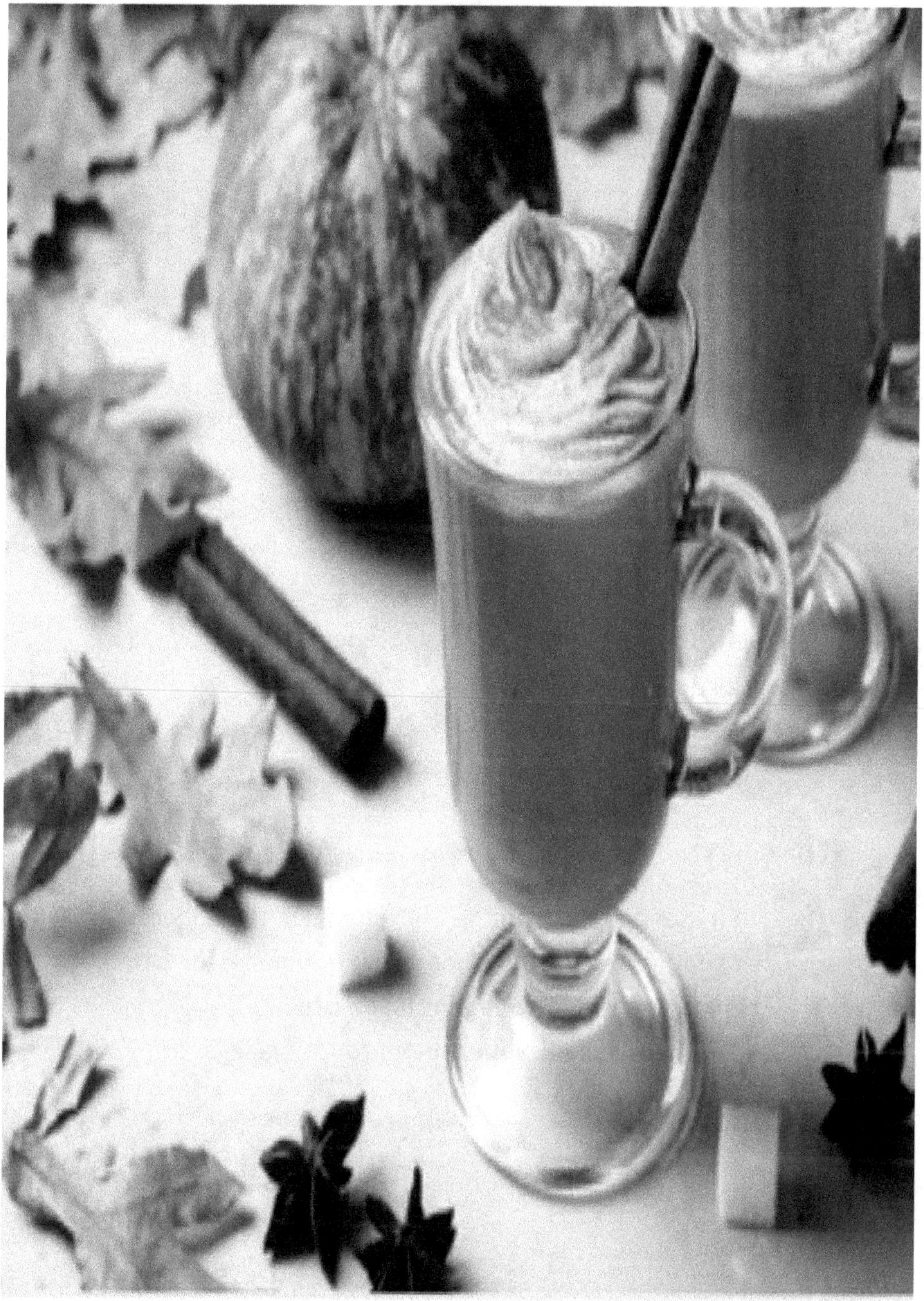

Spicy Pumpkin Frappuccino

Servings: 4

Preparation Time: 5 minutes

Per Serving: Calories: 490 Fat: 9g Protein: 12g Sugar: 11g

Ingredients:

- ½ teaspoon ground cloves
- 2 teaspoons vanilla extract, unsweetened
- 4 teaspoons instant coffee
- 1 teaspoon ground cinnamon
- 4 tablespoons coconut sugar
- ¼ teaspoon nutmeg
- 4 cups almond milk, unsweetened
- 2 cups of ice cubes
- 1 teaspoon ground ginger
- 1/4 teaspoon of all spice

Procedure:

1. First of all, place all the ingredients in the order in a food processor or blender and then pulse for 2 to 3 minutes at high speed until smooth.
2. Then pour the Frappuccino into four glasses and then serve.

Milkshake of Cookie Dough

Servings: 4

Preparation Time: 5 minutes

Per Serving: Calories: 240 Fat: 13g Protein: 21g Sugar: 9g

Ingredients:

- 4 tablespoons cookie dough
- 1 cup almond milk, unsweetened
- 1 teaspoon vanilla extract, unsweetened
- 3 cup almond milk ice cubes
- 10 dates, pitted
- 4 teaspoons chocolate chips

Procedure:

1. Firstly, place all the ingredients in the order in a food processor or blender and then pulse for 2 to 3 minutes at high speed until smooth.
2. Then pour the milkshake into four glasses and then serve with some cookie dough balls.

Hemp & Strawberry Smoothie

Servings: 4

Preparation Time: 5 minutes

Per Serving: Calories: 510 Fat: 18g Protein: 26g Sugar: 12g

Ingredients:

- 2 cups almond milk, unsweetened
- 2 cups of ice cubes
- 1 teaspoon vanilla extract, unsweetened
- 1/4 teaspoon sea salt
- 4 tablespoons maple syrup
- 6 cups fresh strawberries
- 4 tablespoons hemp seeds
- 2 cups vegan yogurt
- 4 tablespoons hemp protein

Procedure:

1. First of all, place all the ingredients in the order in a food processor or blender, except for protein powder, and then pulse for 2 to 3 minutes at high speed until smooth.
2. After that, pour the smoothie into four glasses and then serve.

Blueberry, Hamp and Hazelnut Smoothie

Servings: 4

Preparation Time: 5 minutes

Per Serving: Calories: 195 Fat: 14g Protein: 36g Sugar: 10g

Ingredients:

- 4 tablespoons chocolate hazelnut butter
- 2 small frozen bananas
- 1 1/2 cup almond milk
- 4 tablespoons hemp seeds
- 1 teaspoon vanilla extract, unsweetened
- 3 cups frozen blueberries
- 4 tablespoons chocolate protein powder

Procedure:

1. First, place all the ingredients in the order in a food processor or blender and then pulse for 2 to 3 minutes at high speed until smooth.
2. Then pour the smoothie into four glasses and then serve.

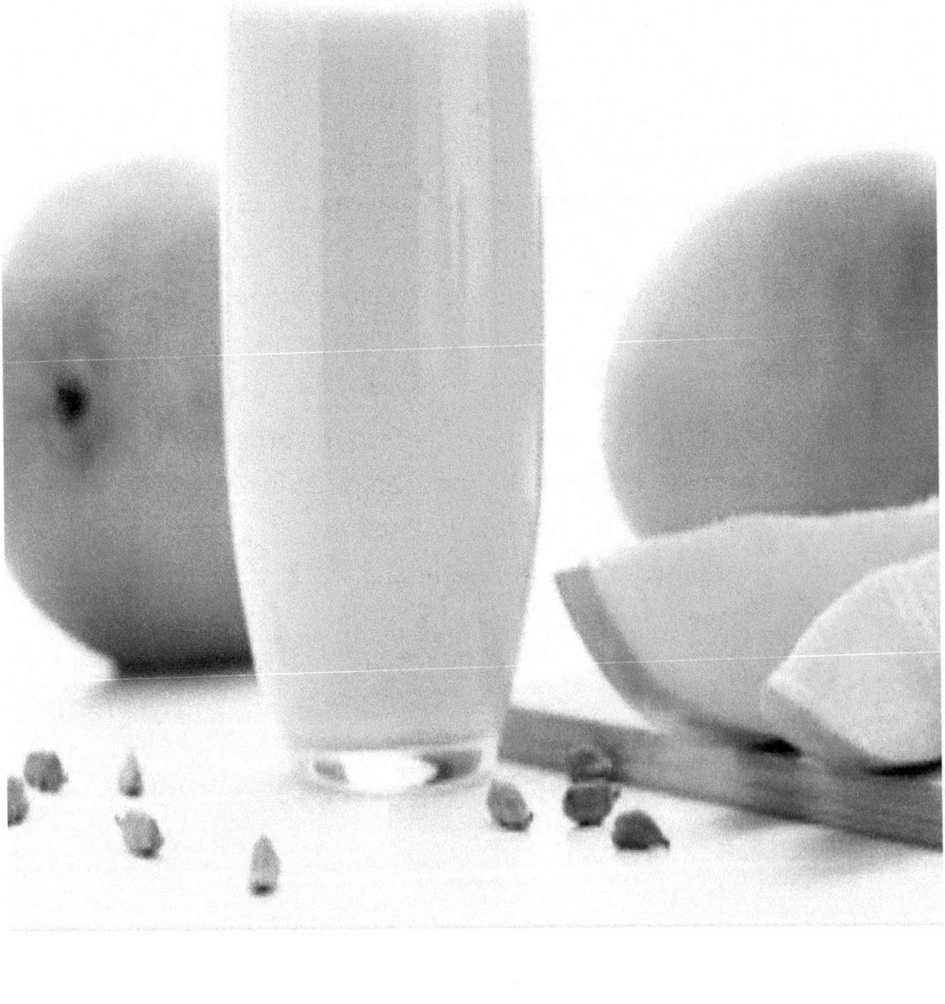

Mango Lassi

Servings: 4

Preparation Time: 5 minutes

Per Serving: Calories: 420 Fat: 12g Protein: 23g Sugar: 13g

Ingredients:

- 2 1/2 cup mango pulp
- 1 teaspoon lemon juice
- 1/2 cup almond milk, unsweetened
- 1/2 cup chilled water
- 2 tablespoons coconut sugar
- 1/4 teaspoon salt
- 2 cups cashew yogurt

Procedure:

1. First, place all the ingredients in the order in a food processor or blender and then pulse for 2 to 3 minutes at high speed until smooth.
2. Then pour the lassi into four glasses and then serve.

Lightning Source UK Ltd.
Milton Keynes UK
UKHW021822160421
382091UK00005B/61